A NATURAL AF

The health of the body h;
Now it's time to tackle t

MW01102075

"Beauty Without Injections" is the face of a new and better world —an unpolluted face that doesn't age.

Using the five, straightforward steps of "F.A.C.E.S. Trade-mark Pending" in "Beauty Without Injections," you'll discover a drug-free, natural way of maintaining ageless beauty.

- Read the incredible truth about the muscle tone of your face.
- Stop the narrowing of your jaw-line—a classic sign of aging.
- Learn the never-before-revealed exercises that will reverse the aging process. (They are not what you think!)
- See how correct posture can create a round and youthful face.
- Control the inner thoughts that can, quite literally, kill you.
- Find out how breathing properly can heal your entire body.
- Take control of your inner hose pipe (blood supply) and water your dry, wilting skin.
- Connect with the extraordinary "computer" (Surgeo and Peaceo) inside of you to stop disease and aging.
- Enjoy huge savings in these tough economic times—95% of these techniques are absolutely free!

...helpful rules for healthy eating, easy-to-follow directions for exercising various parts of the face, and proper posture and breathing techniques ...the author has thoroughly researched her subject - Kirkus Discoveries

Helen E. Day, P.T., C.A.F.C.I., is a qualified physiotherapist, trained in acupuncture. While working on patients with chronic, persistent pain (her specialty) using her developed techniques (a combination of physiotherapy and acupuncture), she found that not only was the pain reduced, but the affected area also looked much younger. By applying these same principles to the face, and by exploring a holistic approach to health in general, she has unlocked the key to ageless health and beauty.

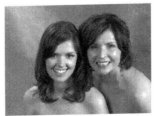

The Author (aged 62) with Daughter
Photo (and front cover photo) by Kim Elsasser

Your skin is your body's largest organ.

Think of it as your finest dress or suit—the one article of clothing that, when you put it on, makes you feel you are the sexiest, hottest, most attractive person in the whole world.

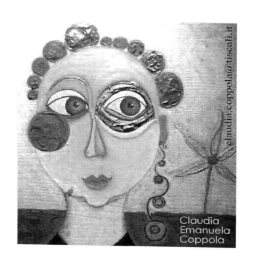

claudia.coppola@tiscali.it

Claudia
Emanuela
Coppola

BEAUTY WITHOUT INJECTIONS

BEAUTY WITHOUT INJECTIONS

HELEN E. DAY P.T., C.A.F.C.I.

Helen E. Day

First Published in 2010 by Helen E. Day, British Columbia, Canada

ISBN: 978-0-9865319-0-3

Typeset by Nom de Plume Writing Services, Suffolk, UK

Available from book stores, and online book retailers, including:
www.amazon.com
www.amazon.ca
www.amazon.co.uk
www.barnesandnoble.com
www.chapters.ca

For information regarding special discounts for bulk purchases, please visit
www.consulteducatetreat.com

Available as an e-book at:
www.ebookit.com
Apple iBookstore
www.amazon.com
www.kobobooks.com
www.bn.com
ebookstore.sony.com
ebooks.google.com
www.diesel-ebooks.com
www.consulteducatetreat.com

To my late father
Dr. Frederic George Day, M.D., Orthopedic Surgeon

To my mother
Alix Roberta Day, Dietician, University of Alberta

To my daughter
Chloe Alexandra Bennett, presently doing her Masters
at University of British Columbia School of Landscape Architecture

They are, and have been, my greatest teachers

Contents – F.A.C.E.S.

F is for Foundation – Chapter One   35

This is not about the make-up you apply to your face. It's about the foundation that supports your skin from the inside. Buildings placed over poor foundations sag over time; so do we!

A is for Acupuncture – Chapter Two   41

Learn about the carefully-guarded, ancient secret of the Chinese royalty that kept their faces young.

and the Autonomic Nervous System   53

This is a "computer" that sits, like a backpack, on either side of your spine. Learn how to keep it balanced so that you build a healthy, sexy face, prevent diseases like high blood pressure and diabetes, and improve your sex life.

C is for Costs – Chapter Three   61

95% of these techniques are free once learned. In these tough economic times, the health and beauty of your face and body can still stay priority number one.

E is for Exercises – Chapter Four   65

The muscles in your face can be your friend, or foe. Learn the exercises that will actually help reduce the effects of aging. (They won't be what you are expecting!)

S is for Skin – Chapter Five   89

Cancer of the skin is on a deadly increase. Learn how to keep your skin clean. Soap and water will not prevent pre-cancerous keratoses. Learn what will. The side benefit is younger-looking skin.

Exercises

Foreword

The author has succeeded in laying out cutting-edge information on how the face ages and, more importantly, on how to stop, maintain and even reverse aging in many cases.

In a concise, straightforward way, the author outlines the major contributors to facial aging and then shows the reader, using pictures and techniques, how to do the repair.

"Beauty Without Injections" is a five-step program for F.A.C.E.S. around the world.

Just as exercise for the body is best started early, the sooner you start this F.A.C.E.S. program, the longer you will be able to maintain your healthy, youthful, facial looks. (It is best started in your teens or twenties.) However, practiced at any age, it will produce dramatic results. Just like body exercise, picking it up when aged 40, 50, 60, 70, 80, or even 90, can produce amazing results in reversing the aging process.

The author only finished the exercise concepts over the last two years, though this book has been in development for the last twelve.

It will amaze you how many of the concepts used are brand new, but, when the author does use older ideas, they are looked at in a fresh new way.

As Albert Einstein said: "There are no ideas so complex that they cannot be explained simply."

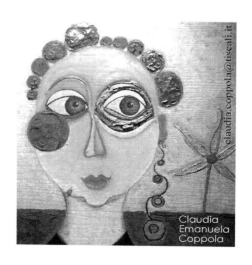

"BEAUTY WITHOUT INJECTIONS"

A BOOK THAT, FOR THE FIRST TIME, TALKS ABOUT
THE HEALTH OF THE FACE AS THE ALL-NATURAL
REPAIR OF THE AGING FACE

A healthy face is a youthful face

A youthful face is round, not long and horsy

A youthful face is sexy

Acknowledgements

I would like to thank the right that I was given, as a woman, to my education. I have always said, "Education is an acquired personal asset that, in this Country, can never be taken away." No amount of learning is ever wasted.

I am so grateful to my patients that, as I developed new techniques to take away their physical pain, the understanding of how to prevent aging of the face evolved. I would like to thank friends and family members who offered sage advice when I was struggling with developing these new concepts and understanding new technology.

My grateful thanks also to the following group of talented professionals who helped in the making of this book. And especially to my wonderful editor, who, with her constant positive reinforcement, sharing the belief that this book will help many, many people, and with her meticulous attention to artistic and editing detail, has made this work a phenomenal success:

Editor, Wendy Toone
Nom de Plume Writing Services Limited, Suffolk, England
mail@ndpwriting.com
www.ndpwriting.com

International Award-Winning Photographer, Kim Elsasser MPA
Kelowna, B.C., Canada
KimsPhotography@shaw.ca
www.kimsphotography.com

Artist, Claudia Emanuela Coppola—Italy
claudia.coppola@tiscali.it
www.facebook.com/claudiaemanuelacoppola

Illustrator, Jennica Hogg
jennica.hogg@gmail.com
www.jajii.deviantart.com

My Personal Journey

What is the Number One thing people hate and fear the most, yet feel they have the least control over?

Aging.

We feel helpless to stop it. We do what we can to slow it down; but we've been conditioned to think we'll never win.

In the old world order, we were expected to accept that our youthful looks would die at middle age. Our destiny was to spend two, three or four decades appearing as wilted flowers; our hearts were heavy and sad because underneath the drooping and sagging, we had lost who we were.

This wilted flower wanted nothing more than to remain youthful and healthy-looking, but was not willing to undergo the insanity of surgery and Botox after becoming aware of the possibly-disastrous side effects.

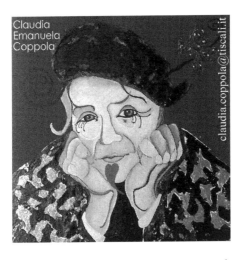

"Beauty Without Injections" is my personal journey as a member of the first year of Baby Boomers to reach 60. Presently 62, I do not use the current popular cosmetic practices and yet I remain youthful in appearance. This appearance I equate with body and facial health.

I wish I could say I have spent my whole life living the five steps of the F.A.C.E.S. program, but I can't. It has been a long, sometimes very painful, process to get where I am today. I sometimes wonder where I would be if I had been able to follow the "Beauty Without Injections" principles from the beginning. Perhaps I would be a newly-evolved human being, because that is what we are supposed to do—evolve. There is a whole new race out there, slowly emerging out of the ashes of the old world.

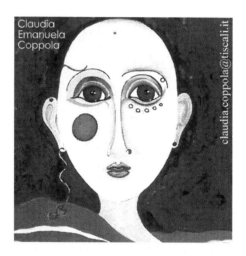

How did I get to this place to write a book on beauty and reveal new concepts about what causes wrinkles and lines on the face?

I was born Helen Elizabeth Day in Edmonton, Alberta, Canada in 1947. My parents were living at this time in Nordegg, Alberta—a small mining town on the eastern slopes of the Rocky Mountains. My father had taken his first position as a doctor after the war, and my mother, who was a University of Alberta graduate dietician, now had two children to look after.

We were to leave shortly after and take the ship "The Queen Elizabeth" to Liverpool, England where my father would take his specialty: Orthopedic Medicine. I was too young to remember the journey, however I'm told I wore a harness on the ship, so I wouldn't go overboard. My older sister and I would wait outside the bar, while my father enjoyed himself. (My mother was pregnant with another sister and very ill.)

My memories only really started when we returned to Edmonton, Alberta. It must have been quite the household—by this time I had three sisters and a brother, in a fairly small house but in the best area of town. I slept in one bedroom with two of my sisters. I remember the most amazing puppet theater we had that was brought back by our grandmother Day from Hawaii. We would put on endless shows, clumsily trying to control the strings with our young, chubby fingers.

There was a lot of fun and laughter; however a darker side had made itself apparent to my young eyes. My father, to handle the stressors of a growing family and, as the best orthopedic surgeon in Edmonton, being responsible for people's lives, was developing an increased dependency on alcohol.

Looking back, it was always what I would call a controlled alcoholism. Through his whole career he always went to work and, as far as I know, was never called up in front of his medical board. But, as is usually the case, it was the family who suffered.

I remember my father's temper from the earliest age. I would instinctively duck whenever I came near him. I don't know how old I was when I was finally able to stop this.

I believe from this came a very strong behavior of always wanting to please.

And yet, mixed with these darker memories, were summers that most children only dream of. We had a summer home at Pigeon Lake, Mameo Beach, Alberta. For several summers (I was probably aged 6 to 10), right after school was out, we would get in the car and ask every 10 minutes if we were there yet.

It was paradise. Dad would stay in Edmonton, working, which eased the tension. We would be set loose in the early morning—only to return for meals—and there would be the gooiest peanut butter sandwiches if we were left alone. Gosh they were good!

Paradise got even bigger when Dad shipped our horses down. The routine was: up at dawn, Mom would have our lunches packed, and off we would head—a rag-tag group of Huckleberry Finns, looking for that pot of gold. Every day was a different adventure.

At about age 11, my parents bought a large farm outside Edmonton. My father was realizing his dearest wish to raise pure-bred Herefords. His summers, as a young boy, were spent with his grandfather, Jock Frame, who was a Member of Parliament for Athabasca, Alberta, Canada.

I became a champion barrel-racer and Gymkhana rider. I don't know where it came from, but put me on a horse and I was a daredevil at everything. I still remember the rush, going at speeds a normal person wouldn't even consider, feeling so at one with my horse. The slightest knee nudge and my beloved companion would respond...This closeness, however, did not spare me from misfortune.

I was coming down to the finish line, pushing my horse faster and faster, when I experienced a surreal sensation. I was floating away from my horse, knowing the ground was coming toward me...

I don't know how long it was before I woke up to my father yelling at me. I know he was terrified. In those days helmets were not worn and I'm told I suffered what would be known today as a head injury.

Physically, I recovered quickly. But mentally, in hindsight, I believe the accident had repercussions.

~

In the following years I was to awaken to my femininity, along with my sisters. You can imagine the chaos with four young women struggling to use the same mirrors (though we had two sinks) as we experimented with make-up, hairdos, etc. My greatest peeve was that my youngest sister would constantly watch me from around the corner of the bathroom door.

Make-up and clothes became everything. I remember poring over the latest Seventeen magazine. The drive for perfection had emerged. I had to be the best at everything. My marks at school in the most part were high, but it did not come easily, and I had to work very hard.

Somewhere during this time-period, my drive for excellence and wanting to please people, took me off course. It was to contribute towards a disorder that I was to suffer from throughout my teens and early adulthood. I would not eat for several days at a time, then I'd gorge. In later years this would become known as Bulimia.

I had to be thin. As happens with sufferers today, I became very depressed. You can imagine the deprivation of nutrients when, for the most part I wouldn't be eating, and when I finally did, I would fill up on junk food. For those of you out there now dealing with this, please know that it *can* end and you can be healed. www.lookingglassbc.com

My despair led me to the deepest depths and I tried to take my life at least 3 times.

I still remember sitting in the emergency ward after I had swallowed a bottle of my father's medication called Stelibid. The effect of the medication was to send my body into spasms. With horror, I could not keep my tongue in my mouth—it was contorting at weird angles.

My sister, who I had called because I did not want to die but didn't know how to live, looked at me and said: "Maybe it's better that you die."

I was told I was very lucky—the spasm would have hit my lungs next and stopped me from breathing.

Another suicide attempt was to slash my wrists, but I used

the razor blade on the inside of my wrist, missing the main radial artery which lies almost on the outside of the wrist, under the thumb. I did this while at University, studying Anatomy, so obviously I didn't really want to die.

And out of my suffering came a deep desire to help other people who are suffering.

Where did my suffering come from? I believe it was a combination of:

1. Genetics—My grandmother, father and mother (all brilliant people) suffered from anxiety and depression to varying degrees.

2. My head injury—The horse riding accident probably took a silent toll on me. I know my compulsive eating started soon after this.

3. A much darker reason would not surface until I was in my forties and fifties. I started to recall a memory of when I was about 6 or 7. We were living in the best part of town, and my best friend and I were playing on a bank overlooking a ravine. Suddenly a stranger came walking out of this ravine and asked us to walk with him, leading us down the embankment. He sexually assaulted me (I was only able to recall this with hypnosis), but I was able to run away and get help for my friend.
   I remember all the police cars, and feeling very much alone. My parents, I'm sure, were hysterical. As was so often the case in those days, I was sat down and told never to talk or think about it again. When I asked my mother "why?" all those years later, she answered: "We thought it was the best thing to do."

I'm very proud of my parents, and certainly don't hold this reaction against them. It was what people did in those times—they covered everything up.

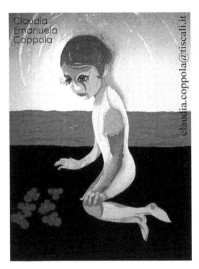

AGING creates suffering

Many years have passed since then. How on earth did I become a normal, balanced individual again? Well, I had periods of being okay, interspersed with being plunged back into the depths of despair. I used to liken it to going along a road—everything would be normal (I'd be getting my weight back to normal), and then suddenly I'd lose sight and direction, and walk right into a utility pole. The result was always deep depression. My weight would balloon, and I'd despise myself.

One day I decided to try running. This was very painful. I immediately got shin splints and I remember my inner thighs would jiggle and rub together. For some reason I didn't give up, and slowly I lost the weight, and my self-esteem started to rise. Running would be a part of my life for the next 25 years.

Finally, the antidepressant, Prozac, came out and, at about the same time, I was introduced to a 12-step program aimed at depression that lasted 6 weeks. I went to a facility located on Vancouver Island, B.C. and it was here that I discovered that I was actually lovable. Before this, my past experiences had forced me to believe I wasn't.

I remember being in a chapel and not realizing that the priest was performing a healing on me. It was incredible. I felt this intense heat penetrate my head, and I started to be aware of something much larger than myself, guiding me. Since then, there have been many times when I've been back in despair and suddenly a warm, invisible cloak wraps itself around me, tugging at my spirit to remind me who I am (almost always when I've remembered to breathe like the wind—gentle and deep).

At the age of 34 I had my first and only child. Prior to her birth I had read an article by the great, redheaded comedian, Lucille Ball, where she'd stated her life only started when she had her children. Before this article I had never wanted children—probably because I was having too much difficulty with myself. It was like a lightening bolt. Having my Chloe gave me a life I never could have comprehended. This little spirit depended totally on me. I was going to be the best Mom I knew how.

I could feel my inner strength really building. Chloe would grow up never seeing her Mom as her former self.

In my forties, I took the first University level of Acupuncture. I would practice on myself, and my strength continued to grow.

Eating healthily also helped. I started haunting the health food stores in my twenties, looking for something to stop my anxieties. I tried everything, going through periods of eating only vegetarian food but always slipping back to "normal" North American eating. After I had my daughter, the pattern would continue—healthy, vegetable-based and then back to North American—but we would eat healthily for long periods. My daughter always says she was raised on healthy fast food—"The Submarine Shop" for example, where I'd get her A sub stacked with lots of veges!

More importantly, my internal dialogue was now becoming so positive. I was turning into the bright, strong person I was always meant to be. My daughter and I can both remember me dropping her off at the Bumble Bee day care, saying: "And what kind of a day are we going to have?" In her little voice, she would always reply: "Just the kind we make up our minds to be."

I remember as a University student studying Physiotherapy, sitting in the cafeteria at the Royal Alex Hospital with one of my classmates, Marlene Davis, and embarking on a mission to keep myself as healthy as possible. Another classmate made a statement which I never forgot and which was a catalyst for the work that has led to this book, "Beauty Without Injections." She said: "Wrinkles are made by moving the face, so I'm not going to express myself anymore." (I wonder how she made out?)

My interest in health, physiotherapy and acupuncture continued, and in 1993 I established my own physiotherapy practice:

www.ConsultEducateTreat.com

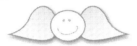

Then, in 1998, at the age of 51, I woke up to the fact that my face was showing my age. Here I was, a Baby Boomer, the largest, most cohesive and powerful group this world has ever seen, and yet even we could not stop the assault of advancing years.

I was wiser than I'd ever been, capable of almost anything, and yet every morning my aging face stared back at me. I was intelligent enough to know that there had to be something out there besides a quick cosmetic fix. I was constantly looking at western and complementary practices for the health of the body; so now was the time to address the face.

At about this same time, I also decided to specialize my physiotherapy practice to focus on persistent, or chronic, pain. (Most physiotherapists deal with acute problems such as broken wrists, low back strain, tendonitis, etc., which tend to heal in a set time-frame.)

I could see that with the aging Baby Boomers, pain that did *not* go away in a set time period was going to become a huge problem. And indeed, today it is.

As I focused on developing techniques to help heal this "tough" pain, I observed an interesting and unexpected phenomenon:

AS THE PATIENT'S AFFECTED BODY PART HEALED, IT ALSO APPEARED YOUNGER!

From this exciting observation, a question started to permeate my daytime thinking:

Could it be possible to retain a vibrant and young appearance well into our old age?

This question would not leave me alone, and ultimately, it produced "Beauty Without Injections"—a program of empowerment for all men and women.

Taking the best from eastern and western techniques and traditions, "Beauty Without Injections" uses well-known principles, mostly from physiotherapy and acupuncture, and demonstrates them in five simple steps. These steps can leave you looking 10 to 20 years younger, and will enhance the wellness of your entire body.

~

Life is a series of choices. It's the choices we make that determine how the next part of our life plays out. Sometimes we make good choices; sometimes bad ones.

Looking back, I can see how the health and beauty choices I have made over the years have played their part in the road I have traveled.

After years of adult acne, I consulted a doctor who recommended dermabrasion. The process, at that time, was to be given a general anesthetic, have the entire top layer of the facial skin taken off, and then exist on a cocktail of painkillers, sleeping pills and tranquilizers for several days. I decided against it. This would have been a bad choice for me as it was very invasive (and later would prove unnecessary).

However, at about the same time (in my early thirties) I read about the discovery of "Retin-A" while leafing through a Vogue magazine. I remember seeing a pair of old rats with smooth, young skin, and was very impressed. I went to a dermatologist and I have used Retin-A, off and on, ever since. This was a good choice for me, as it is non-invasive, and, over time, it has taken away the marks of the acne.

Next I read (again in a magazine) that the best way to avoid wrinkles was to have surgery before the wrinkles started. So off I went to have the first (and last) surgical procedure on my face. Several weeks after the operation, my father (the orthopedic surgeon), took the stitches out, but when I got home, I noticed my lower eyelid had contracted outward, showing the inner white. I went back as an outpatient, my one-year-old daughter at my side. I had to keep her entertained by dangling car keys, while my scar tissue was dealt with under local anesthetic. It had never occurred to me that surgery might not be 100% effective.

A few years later, still concerned by my appearance, I saw the services of a local Esthetician advertised. European-trained, this specialist guaranteed to take years off my looks. I had traveled extensively during my twenties, and had always been impressed at how well-groomed European women were—especially the French. It seemed taken for granted over there that young women would follow their mothers and start to look after their skin at an early age.

So in I went, and soon I was talking to a beautiful, older Hungarian woman. I was probably convinced to go ahead by her appearance alone.

I took the appointment for the next Friday and was told it would only take a few days for me to recover.

All I remember was sitting in a chair, a sudden blur of pain, the smell of burning flesh and an overwhelming desire to run. A huge fan blowing air on my face was my only solace. When it was finally over, the Hungarian lady walked me to my car and said she would call.

I woke up the next day to a face that was crusty white. (I was later to learn that I'd been given a chemical peel.) It took two weeks before I could finally return to work—but the results were wonderful! All vestiges of sun damage had gone…however, I couldn't help wondering what could have happened if she hadn't been so well trained.

My next foray into the maintenance of my looks was one of those fated occurrences that would seal my fate for the course I was to take for the rest of my career.

I read about a Chiropractor who was extolling the virtues of acupuncture face-lifts. The fact that acupuncture was non-invasive was a major selling point to me. Non-invasive meant no pain, no trauma, and no possibility of things going wrong. I saw some very impressive before and after pictures, booked a series of appointments, and the results were amazing on me. This was an excellent choice, and for the next several years I continued with the acupuncture treatment and maintained a healthy lifestyle— running regularly 3–4 times a week and eating properly.

In 1991, an acupuncture course was offered for the first time in North America at a professional level. Aimed at physiotherapists, doctors and dentists, I qualified to go as a physiotherapist, and, after graduating, I opened my own practice—occasionally performing facial acupuncture on myself. The results were always the same: I looked younger and felt better. I would notice better circulation, tightened skin and clearer eyes.

As the years went by and my daughter left for college, I went through what can only be described as the "empty nest" syndrome. I started on a misguided route of looking for other ways to enhance my looks.

For two more years I tried everything short of surgery. I had Botox around my eyes and ignored the voice that told me of the possible complications. I went in regularly to have my lips pumped up with Restylane. (I finally figured out the appeal of the overly-filled lips—they represent the engorged labia of the female sexual organs. So the more filled they are, the more you look ready for sexual activity.) Needless to say I received a lot of interest, but not the kind I wanted.

Coming to my senses with the above realization, and also spending far too much money at $400 a pop every two months, I could see how addictive this was to women who wanted to remain young-looking and attractive to men. When I finally went in to say I would not be returning, the nurse told me she admired me. "Not many women can stop once they have started," she said.

We all have choices to make about the way we treat our body AND FACE, inside and out.

Regular choices can range from invasive surgery to expensive moisturizers. But I now choose to use the five steps of "Beauty Without Injections" to keep me youthful.

~

I always enjoy the quote by ADELLE DAVIS, nutritionist and author:

> *"As I see it, everyday you do one of two things build health or produce disease in yourself."*

Our health care system does not emphasize prevention; we are too busy fixing what could have been prevented. It is this preventative aspect that is missing in our culture and it is precisely what is needed for the optimal health of our body and looks.

As a physiotherapist, I know that physiotherapy has always stood for prevention. For decades, physiotherapists have looked after this in the human body. They have an advanced understanding of how the body moves, what keeps it from moving well and how to restore mobility.

It is my job to promote, prevent, rehabilitate and cure the human body while educating my patients.

Prevention and management of physical impairments (which includes aging), is imperative for health and beauty.

Combining the advancements in the western world with eastern philosophy has created the new paradigm of our new and aging world. Our population is aging. The last century has seen vast changes in Canadian, American and European Union populations—a steady decrease in fertility (with the notable exception of the Baby Boomers), a decrease in the death rate and an increase in life expectancy. In 1971, there were 7 people of working age (20–64) to every senior citizen. By 2006, this had gone down to 5. And it is predicted that by 2056 (when the first Baby Boomers will be in their 100s, if they are still here), there will be only 2 working people to every senior. We must start to take responsibility for our own health so that we can be in a position to help the less fortunate. (Plus, the largest gift we can give our loved ones is not to get sick.)

So far though, according to statistics, this responsibility for our own health is not happening.

Baby Boomers are not making a good job of aging, and, unless there is a change, the major implications are: an ever-increasing drain on our health service, a massive push on pharmaceuticals and a huge increase in cosmetic practices.

The one common denominator of 1/3 of the population of Canada and 80 million Americans is that they are aging fast and they are not doing it well. They are more obese and inactive than those ahead of them:

Statistics Canada 2008 www.statcan.gc.ca

When you combine those who are overweight and those who are obese, 58.6% of men and 43.5% of women are at increased health risk because of their excess weight.

In Canada, 27% of deaths are caused by cancer. Heart disease is next, at 26.6%, with cerebrovascular (brain dysfunctions like stroke) coming in third at 7.4%. (Stats Canada.)

In the United States, the stats are similar, with heart disease at 28.5%, cancer at 22.8% and cerebrovascular disease at 6.7%. (US Census Bureau.)

Evidence continues to mount that, to some extent, these are preventable diseases, and studies have shown that being in good health reduces your chances of encountering them.

So where are North Americans placing their health dollars if not to prevent their own diseases?

In many instances, disposable income is put towards looking good on the outside (and this includes homes and cars as well as Botox and fillers), rather than maintaining their health on the inside.

[1] The American Academy of Cosmetic Surgery (2008, March 14) reported that among patients treated, 80% were women and 20% were men. Of the procedures performed, 23% were surgical, with the remaining 77% being non-surgical procedures.

[2] In 2007 there were nearly 11.7 million surgical and non-surgical cosmetic procedures performed in the United States. Surgical procedures accounted for nearly 18% of the total.

- There were 2,775,176 procedures of Botox injection, and 1,448,716 procedures involving hyaluronic acid.
- Women had nearly 10.6 million cosmetic procedures—91% percent of the total.
- 46% of the procedures were done on people aged 35–50 (5.4 million); 25% were performed on people aged 51–64; and 21% were performed on people aged 19–34. The 65s-and-overs accounted for 6% of the procedures; and those aged

1   *Statistics courtesy of the American Society for Aesthetic Plastic Surgery*

2   *Statistics courtesy of Medicard Finance*

18-and-younger comprised less than 2%.

- Since 1997, there has been a 457% increase in the total number of cosmetic procedures. Surgical procedures have increased by 114%, and non-surgical procedures have increased by 754%.

We spend a pittance on our health compared to the millions we spend on beauty enhancement like surgery, cosmetics, lotions, oils, creams and clothing.

In order to understand how this book will benefit you, we need to adjust our perspective on youth, aging and health in general.

It's true that none of us is getting any younger, and the powers behind the "beauty marketing machine" won't let us forget it. In our world, the media bombards us with visions of beautiful people—the famous, the rich, the talented, the privileged—and all of them looking great. Advertisements and commercials have these same beautiful people pitching us on how they maintain their youthful appearance, usually through lotions, creams or a medical procedure. Tabloid TV and magazines feed us information on who has had what procedure done.

Very few promote health as a means to beauty and a youthful appearance. And the reason is because, once you've learned it, it's free. There is no need to buy refills, return for another procedure, or stock up on the latest cream.

Your face is essentially the same as the rest of your body—if you keep yourself healthy, you will not only feel better and younger, but you will *look* younger too. If you think of your arm for instance—let's say the muscles, circulation, nerves and bones aren't in harmony—your inability to move properly makes you look older. Likewise, if you try to walk with lower back strain, you'll bend over, shuffle, a painful grimace on your face—not the look of youth!

With the F.A.C.E.S. program in "Beauty Without Injections" you will learn:

- That stress is the number one cause of aging, and that there is a little "computer" in your body that controls stress. It is actually a "Tree of Life" in your body, called the Autonomic Nervous System. This poorly understood system is completely out of control in most people, contributing not only to illness but also to the aging process. Here you will learn how to keep it balanced.
- That sun damage only *contributes* to the underlying cause of wrinkles. Learn, finally, what causes a wrinkle.
- That aging of the face is not caused by *loss* of muscle tone, but actually by *increased* muscle tone, covered by sagging skin. Traditional facial exercises only make this worse!
- That with aging comes the narrowing of the jaw due to stiffening jaw joints, which causes the skin to sag. Face-lifts try to correct this, but excess skin is just pulled over a narrowed jaw line. Learn the exercises that will keep the jaw joint flexible.
- That dark circles and bags under the eyes can be corrected by releasing the jaw muscles (masseter, temporalis, etc.).
- That jowls and double chins can be related to faulty posture.
- That poor posture is reflected in the entire state of the face. Learn how good posture creates a youthful and round face, rather than a long and horsy one.

By following the five, simple steps (F.A.C.E.S.) in "Beauty Without Injections," you can retain your looks and health even into your 100s.

It starts right here, right now, with you.

Chapter One – F.A.C.E.S.

F is for Foundation

A healthy foundation is a must if this program is to be effective for you.

This starts with being under good medical advice and *following* that advice for any medical condition. (Supervision can be provided by a medical doctor or naturopathic physician, or both, as is the case for many today.)

Proper rest is also essential.

And then of course, there's diet. There are books galore out there that cover healthy diets, so find the one that's right for you. This could be an "allergy" diet—gluten or dairy free—or one that follows the glycemic index. To know which diet is the right one for you, keep a food diary and make a note of how you feel after eating certain things. It doesn't matter if something tastes great—if you feel sluggish the next day or feel ill afterwards, it isn't good for you!

Consult a dietician, naturopath, physician or doctor of traditional medicine, and work together to develop a plan for healthy eating that suits you personally. Then follow it daily.

Two Basic Rules For Healthy Eating

Perimeter-Only Shopping

You may have already heard about the perimeter rule, but it bears repeating. Only shop the perimeter areas of the grocery stores. That way, you avoid the packaged and processed foods. This rule also applies to health food stores. Yes the food is healthier in health food stores, but those baked (not fried) chips are still processed, and more than likely will have added salt.

Know Your Food Source
If you have your own garden, you are blessed, for you know the soil and everything that goes into and onto your produce. For those without the time or garden space, shop the farmers' markets in the summer, and buy organic, when available, in the winter months.

Whenever possible, avoid any food whose origin isn't easily traced. Learn who your local producers are for dairy products, meats and vegetables. If you can find out where your food is coming from, you'll not only be wiser, you'll be healthier too.

Most cities have businesses that will source out locally grown, organic foods. Shop there yourself, or if you haven't the time, find a delivery service whereby fresh produce is delivered to your door on a weekly or bi-weekly basis.

Everyone complains about the cost of organic food—but here's a tip:

Some businesses that deliver to your home will offer surplus produce, once a week (usually on a Saturday), out of their warehouse, at just above cost.

A web site that has good information:
http://www.certifiedorganic.bc.ca/aboutorganic/whybuy.php
Also, even if you can only buy one or two organic items, it's a start.

[Remember, the 60,000 mostly repetitive thoughts you have daily profoundly affect your health much more than what you ingest. The body/mind connection means that your thoughts can literally be a poison or the antidote. Just think of the cost savings you can make if you control what goes through your mind with visualization etc.]

If you don't have a budget for strictly organic foods, read the stickers. Some countries have very lax guidelines when it comes to the pesticides used on their produce. Don't be complacent about your food; learn where it comes from and what the food safety practices are in the country of origin.

For example, according to government officials, 39 of the 928 pesticides registered and in use in Chile are on the United Nations' list of pesticides prohibited or severely restricted by governments. So those grapes might look really tasty and healthy—but are they? Educate yourself and be food smart.

Surprisingly, the David Suzuki Foundation report, "the food we eat," notes that unlike other countries, Canada has not set stringent "maximum residue levels" for many pesticides, though the government is currently revisiting this issue.

For instance, strawberries laced with carbofuran are not allowed in Europe or Australia (where the maximum residue level is 0 parts per million), but Canada and the U.S. will accept them, as their maximum residue level (MRL) is 0.4 and 0.5 respectively.

Also, learn the difference between "grain-fed," "free-range" and "organic." A chicken may be free-range but if it is munching down insecticide-dusted bugs, those chemicals will end up in your eggs and in the meat that you eat.

A healthy diet is the cornerstone of a healthy body and youthful appearance. Food fuels our body, and the old adage "garbage in—garbage out" is never truer than it is today as we become surrounded by fast-food restaurants on every corner.

Finding a healthy way to eat may not be easy, but the results are well worth it.

You can check out your food guide online—prepare an outline of healthy foods that you like, and base your eating choices around them.

A good way to keep to your healthy diet is to spend time in advance, preparing your food for the week ahead. For example, take an hour to wash a week's worth of vegetables. Or prepare vegetable salads the evening before. The more organized you are, the less likely you are to slip up and hit the drive thru!

Fruits and vegetables are highly important for good health—

and that includes good pH health. A balanced pH is where the proper level of alkalinity is maintained in our cells. Our bodies are alkaline by design. An imbalance of alkalinity creates an environment where bacteria, yeast and other unwanted organisms rapidly multiply. All fields of health and healing recognize that pH (or the acid-alkaline balance), is the most important part of a balanced and healthy body, and that it's crucial to cellular health. Foods like asparagus, beets, broccoli, berries, grapes, grapefruit, as well as eggs, cinnamon, garlic and seeds are excellent for balancing your pH. Add apple cider vinegar to your diet, and drink green tea.

Put all your alkaline fruit and vegetables in a blender drink. Here's one I like to use:

Take a chunk of ginger;
¼ cup of organic lemon juice or apple cider vinegar;
2 cups of kale, broccoli, beet greens, dandelion greens, or whatever you happen to have in your fridge right now, even salad greens;
Banana, berries;
Stevia (herbal sweetener);
Add filtered water;
Blend and enjoy!

I make this up in the a.m. and it is always gone by the p.m.

What I find today is a great discrepancy of "alkaline to acid" lists. So use your common sense; if it is green, it is probably alkaline.

Have you noticed when you are given flowers—be they potted plants or bouquets— how the green parts always last the longest? They are also probably alkaline. Therefore, taking your greens will help *you* last longer.

Finally, use Himalayan crystal salt, which contains up to 84 elements (see www.heartfeltliving.com).

These are just a few of the foods you can add to, or increase in, your diet to help restore or maintain your health.

The very wise choice of zero tolerance to chemicals in our food and "junk food" has also been moving into other areas of our lives. Did you know that the average woman uses at least 17 known carcinogens daily in her make-up, hair products, etc.?

People are increasingly adopting a zero tolerance approach to chemicals in their shampoos, deodorants, laundry soaps, etc. And this is also a growing trend in cosmetics.

Skin was once thought to be the ultimate barrier between preventing toxins from entering our bodies. But we now know that these deadly chemicals can, and do, pass through the skin and enter the blood stream.

A list of cosmetic ingredients to consider avoiding can be found at www.organicmakeup.ca. This website was set up by Lori Stryker, the founder of Toronto-based "Organic Make-up Company", to educate the public.

Some chemical-free cosmetic suppliers:
- Physicians Formula's new organic wear line—found at Wal-Mart and drug stores.
- The German company "Lavera"—found at London Drugs, The Bay and Rexall.

Again, people are often put off by the cost, but simply buying only one item at first and then slowly replacing pieces as your old cosmetic runs out, works well. Remember, the more we buy these chemical-free products, the more the competition will grow and the prices will come down.

Did you know there is a natural alternative to conventional deodorant? Mineral salts form a natural barrier against odor-causing bacteria. The plus, plus side to using one of these natural deodorants is that it will last for years. It is sold under the label "Natural Fresh Deodorant Crystal," and I last came across it at

"Superstore."

Also, good old vinegar has been used as a deodorant for centuries!

One final foundation tip: have www.realage.com e-mail you daily with advice on how to stay healthy.

Chapter Two – F.A.C.E.S.

A is for Acupuncture
(F.A.C.E.S. Acupuncture)
& the Autonomic Nervous System

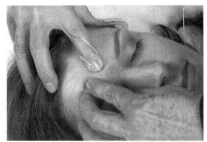

By Kim Elsasser

Once you understand F.A.C.E.S. Acupuncture—a combination of Acupuncture, C-Shape and Scrabbling—and the Autonomic Nervous System, you will be well on your way to retaining your youthful looks and health.

F.A.C.E.S. Acupuncture (F.A.)

Over the past twenty years there has been a slow blending of eastern and western medical practices in North America. A large proportion of the general population knows there are techniques and medicines from both practices that can help them, and many people are moving more and more to the use of naturopaths etc. This new paradigm is one of the keys to looking and feeling healthier.

Imagine if you will, that you are at a lavish smorgasbord. As you gaze down the table you are amazed by the array of different foods presented there. There are foods from around the world—

almost no country or nationality is left out. The interesting thing is, today's informed consumer probably knows a little bit about most of these foods, and modern-day health enthusiasts are able to pick the nutritional best from a global market.

In this book, "Beauty Without Injections," I extend this cosmopolitan trend to changing the aging of the face—for there is a rapidly-growing group of people who want to diminish the appearance of aging without relying on the typically western practices of surgery, Botox and injectables.

Treatments like acupuncture go back thousands of years in China. In the new Stone Age, bian stones were found. These stones were heated and then applied to special points on the body. From there it was a slow transition to the use of bones, then bamboo and finally to today's disposable, stainless steel needles.

How was this amazing technique discovered? Legend tells of a Chinese warrior, who, during battle, was struck by a spear in the middle of his right shin. The warrior had been suffering from a painful left shoulder for many years, but after being hit with the spear in his shin, the pain in his shoulder disappeared. That particular point on his body is now known as "Stomach 38" and is known for its healing properties to the shoulder on the opposite side.

Acupuncture became the main healing method in many ancient civilizations. The use of acupuncture to improve the appearance of the face remained a closely-guarded secret of the Chinese royalty, and it was only after the Communist takeover that these secrets were revealed to the general public.

To understand how F.A.C.E.S. Acupuncture works, you need to know that:

1. Your skin is your body's largest organ

Think of your skin as your finest dress or suit—the one article of clothing that, when you put it on, makes you feel you are the hottest, sexiest, most attractive person in the whole world.

The clothing fits well if the body is healthy. But if the body is unhealthy, the skin will fit too tightly or hang too loosely.

To have healthy skin, yes, you need to nourish it on the outside, but you also need to nourish it from the inside.

As the body is injured, ages or goes under stress, the underlying muscles shrink and tighten. On the inside, the muscles shrink, and on the outside the skin loosens. The shrinking of the muscles also traps nerves and blood vessels that supply the skin.

The muscles have now become short, taut bands with knots (tender trigger points which serve as acupuncture points) in them.

[You can learn more about trigger points and taut bands by reading Doctors Janet Travell and David Simons's highly-respected, two-volume medical textbook, "Myofascial Pain & Dysfunction: The Trigger Point Manual."]

So, contrary to popular opinion, aging facial muscles are actually taut and "over toned." Traditional facial exercises designed to tighten the underlying muscles and improve sagging skin, only make things worse!

2. Muscles, when they age or are injured, slowly start to turn "wooden"

Aging muscles begin to lack the ability to heal themselves.

During acupuncture, a super-thin, sterilized, stainless steel needle is inserted into the trigger point (the muscle knot), and the body initiates a cascade of reactions aimed at repair and restoration at the point of "trauma" (the needle-point at the tender trigger point).

Hence the aging tissue, muscle and collagen begin to heal/repair. The wood (fibrotic tissue) turns back to soft tissue.

F.A.C.E.S. Acupuncture—What To Expect

This could be one of the most profoundly relaxing experiences of your life.

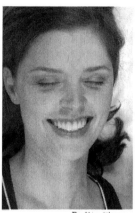

By Kim Elsasser

When you embark on a series of F.A.C.E.S. Acupuncture treatments, you should feel no unpleasant side effects if you are in the hands of a qualified practitioner. There may, however, be slight bruising if you are prone to bruising.

F.A.C.E.S. Acupuncture (F.A.) treats the face *and the entire body.* The face is a micro system, with each area of the face representing an organ in the body. For instance, the area under the eye represents the kidney.

This concept is easier to grasp if you understand reflexology, where practitioners apply deep, sustained pressure to a specific area of the foot. This pressure promotes healing elsewhere in a specific part of the body.

With F.A.C.E.S. Acupuncture (F.A.), a healing and wellness happens in the face, body and organs simultaneously.

F.A. not only affects muscles, but also the connective tissues that surround the muscles in your face. Stimulating connective tissue through F.A. improves circulation and oxygenation, and also encourages lymph drainage and the elimination of toxins. This in turn helps to soften wrinkles in the skin above the muscles, while relaxing the muscles below.

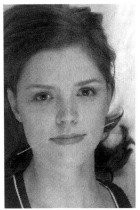

By Kim Elsasser

Your face softens and appears younger. After just a few treatments, your friends will tell you how rested you look. Your wrinkles won't have disappeared, but their appearance will be less deep. You'll notice less loose skin on your face because the muscles underneath will be healthy and relaxed. You'll also have a soft glow to your skin, because when muscles relax, blood and nerve transmission is enhanced.

Before & After Photos

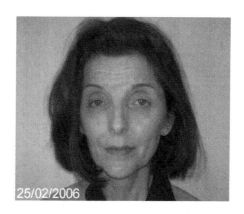

52-year-old woman

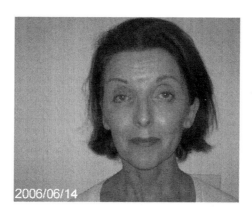

*After following the 5-step F.A.C.E.S. program,
including 12 sessions of F.A./Scrabbling/C-Shape*

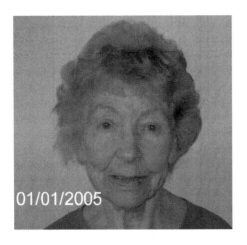

90-year-old woman

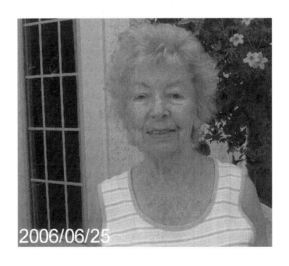

*After following the 5-step F.A.C.E.S. program,
including 12 sessions of F.A./Scrabbling/C-Shape*

Most individuals under 30 need only practice the 5 steps. Over 30, it is highly recommended that you have a series of 12 sessions of F.A.C.E.S. Acupuncture (smokers can expect 20 sessions or more), and then practice the 5 maintenance steps. (Please contact the author at www.ConsultEducateTreat.com to set up some appointments.)

Further F.A. treatments will be required when you start to lose the round look of youth and redevelop the long, "horsy" look of aging, but your next experience will be amazing because the body doesn't forget acupuncture and will respond very quickly. Also you can extend the effect between treatments for longer— if not eliminate the need for more treatment altogether—by performing the exercises outlined in Chapter Four.

You may need additional F.A. if you undergo extreme mental or physical stress in your life, but you'll find that acupuncture will pull your entire body out of the trauma.

Choosing a Practitioner

Be very careful when choosing a practitioner. The popularity of F.A.C.E.S. Acupuncture is increasing, as people search for alternative ways to maintain their looks. This will mean that people without proper training will be trying to get into the field.

Research their credentials, ask for references and thoroughly research their background before making your choice.

The success of these treatments is dependent upon finding a good, qualified practitioner; but, even more importantly, it depends on how well you look after your own health.

In order to achieve maximum results from F.A. you must:

- Eat a nutritious and balanced diet.
- Be a non-smoker—if you are a smoker it will take an additional 8 to 12 treatments to see an improvement.
- Not abuse drugs or alcohol.
- Practice the 5 steps of the F.A.C.E.S. program.

- Follow your heart's desire, and be involved in the things that you love.

Will you still see a result if your foundation is less than ideal? The answer is, yes. Because acupuncture heals, whatever your level of health. But the healthier you are, the better the outcome.

One of the ways acupuncture heals is by creating *balance*, through a process called "HOMEOSTATIS". This word means "a state of balance (equilibrium), or a tendency to reach that, metabolically, within a cell or organism."

Acupuncture restores body balance, creating inner peace and tranquility, which in turn promotes healing (as healing only happens in a relaxed state).

Out of Balance   *Balanced*

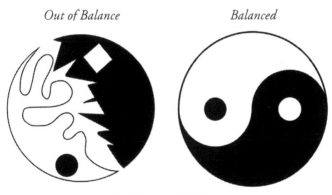

Yin & Yang Balls by Jennica Hogg

So often our systems are drastically out of balance. We need to strive for peaceful balance between our "yin" and "yang" yet the poor yin/yang ball is so sick in today's society.

If you can't afford the cost of a F.A.C.E.S. Acupuncture series, there are some basic F.A. exercises that you can perform yourself, in the comfort of your own home. (Or, if you have a partner or friend that you feel safe and secure with, why not work on each other?)

Home Instructions for F.A.C.E.S. Acupuncture

1. Lie down in a peaceful, quiet room, wearing loose and comfortable clothing.

2. Apply gentle, sustained pressure, for 1½ to 3 minutes, to the acupuncture points in the illustration on Page 52. (Work on both sides of your face at the same time.) Once you feel a gentle relaxation, move on to the next point. The light release under your fingers is hard to pick up at first—it's a feeling of going down a slide—a soft whoosh. But you'll soon be so good at it, especially when you think loving thoughts.

   When you have finished, try the "body" acupuncture points described.

3. Follow this with the exercises outlined in Chapter Four:
   - Page 72   Scrabbling.
   - Page 73   C-Shape.

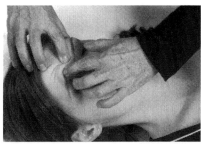

By Kim Elsasser

   - Page 75   Connective Tissue Stretch.
   - Page 86   Breathing—You should perform deep and slow, diaphragmatic breathing as you carry out the sustained pressure routine outlined in Step 2 above. Each

time you breathe out, you will feel the acupuncture point relax a little.

With each complete breath, know that you are healing yourself. (With each *incomplete* breath, know that you are actually destroying yourself.)

- Page 80   Jaw Exercises.
- Page 84   Posture.

4. Now that you have treated the inside, it's time to treat the outside and apply a facial masque. No need to hurry out and buy an expensive one—I have used the following recipe since my teens:

Take one free-range (no pesticides in food) egg. Crack open and separate the white from the yolk.

- If you are under 30, with a more oily skin, use the egg white.

- If you are over 30, use the egg yolk.

- If your skin is very dry, add a small amount of organic olive oil.

Pat on face. Have a good laugh at yourself in the mirror, let it dry (10 minutes maximum), then wash off.

Acupuncture Points

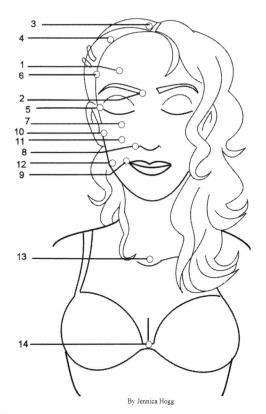

By Jennica Hogg

Location of Points:
1. GB14—1-finger breadth above middle of eyebrow.
2. YINTANG—Inner corner of eyebrow.
3. DU23—1-finger breadth into hair-line.
4. ST8—Corner of forehead.
5. GB1—Depression beside eye.
6. GB6—2 inches above the ears.
7. ST1—Under eyeball.
8. LI20—Top of groove to mouth, beside nose.
9. ST4—Beside corner of mouth.
10. ST7—In depression in front of ear.
11. ST3—Below eye.
12. ST6—On mound of muscle with teeth clenched.
13. REN22—Top of breast bone.
14. REN17—Between breasts.

Body Points:

SP6—4 fingers up from the inside of the ankle bone.

ST36—1-finger breadth below the outside of the knee joint.

LI4—On the mound between the 1st and 2nd finger.

PE6—Inside & 3 fingers up from wrist joint.

REN6—1 inch below belly button.

Autonomic Nervous System

In about the year 2000, while studying a diagram of the Autonomic Nervous System (A.N.S.) which I had seen a few hundred times before, I suddenly saw it for the first time.

Its various branches looked like a tree, with its roots coming out of the spinal cord.

It was at this point that I named it "THE TREE OF LIFE."

The Autonomic Nervous System is not the nerve system that makes your arms and legs move. It is a totally different nerve system that controls all the body's disease processes, and consequently the aging process.

The Autonomic Nervous System (A.N.S.) is the ultimate Tree of Life.

Think of it as a huge computer, sitting on either side of the spinal column like an elongated backpack, capable of balancing all our body systems.

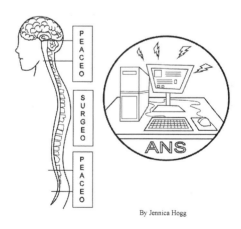

By Jennica Hogg

We have "SURGEO", or the Sympathetic Nervous System, emerging from the back spine bones (thoracic and lumbar).

Surgeo kicks into high gear when the body is under stress.

And "PEACEO", or the Parasympathetic Nervous System, emerging from the upper cervical nerves and tailbone.

Peaceo works to calm things down after a Surgeo episode.

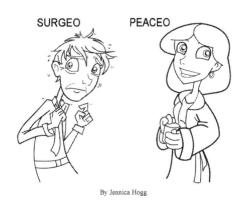

SURGEO   PEACEO

By Jennica Hogg

For the most part, just like your home computer, the A.N.S. (Tree of Life) works well on its own. Unfortunately though, when the A.N.S. computer develops a virus or glitch, there isn't a "body" computer technician to come out and fix it, and we can't just buy a new one.

All escalating human illnesses can be linked to the malfunctioning of the A.N.S. body computer. Medical doctors can only provide drugs to alleviate/mask the problem or treat a small part of it.

The A.N.S. is the body's master balancer or engine, and it needs to run smoothly in order for us to stay healthy and youthful-looking. This engine, in the vast majority of North Americans, is quite simply overheating and blowing up.

The tell-tale signs are all there: steam pouring out of our radiators (high blood pressure), smoke gushing from the tail pipe (irritable bowel syndrome), all tubes to the engine rotting (artery and vein disease), and a broken and dragging tail pipe (impotence).

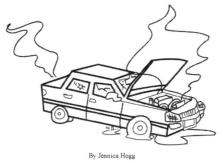

By Jennica Hogg

Diseases such as diabetes, high blood pressure, liver disease, arterial disease, colitis, irritable bowel syndrome, Crohn's disease and, yes, even aging, are the result of an imbalanced Autonomic Nervous System.

And especially for men—erectile dysfunction:

When a man is under long-term stress (or even if he is just worried about his performance in bed), Surgeo raises its ugly head and blood moves inwards, away from the skin and the penis. In order to have a healthy erection, Peaceo is needed to send the blood flowing back to the extremities. (Note: The same problem affects a woman's clitoral erection.)

To relieve stress and encourage Peaceo, and also to prevent premature ejaculation, focus on proper breathing during sex as outlined on Page 86.

Try to imagine a world with no illnesses or pain. Doctors Deepak Chopra and Andrew Weil, among many others, have always maintained that it *is* possible to live a healthy and robust life, and when the universal life-force calls us back home, to experience a very quick and pain-free demise.

So what have these people done to be so blessed? They have achieved knowledge of the workings of their master computer.

They have taken the long journey back to experiencing body balance.

Repairing the Autonomic Nervous System

The good news is, there are natural methods available to help repair the Tree of Life.

Acupuncture, when performed by a qualified, knowledgeable practitioner, is a good start. The Chinese knew, thousands of years ago, that there must be a balance of yin and yang. Good health, peace and decreased aging are achieved when yin (Parasympathetic) and yang (Sympathetic) are in balance.

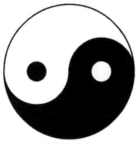

By Jennica Hogg

Most of the eastern practices, such as yoga, meditation, qi gong and tai chi, help restore body balance. In fact, any exercise like running, kick-boxing, rollerblading, a walk in the hills or a walk down the street, is the perfect way to ensure your continued health.

Don't forget the little things too, like laughter, good healing thoughts directed toward yourself, doing a kind deed, and, of course, eating healthy foods. In fact, anything that brings peace to your system, and that is non addictive, is a step in the right direction. As a child you may recall rolling down a hillside and laughing with glee, or lying in a meadow and gazing up at fluffy clouds in a perfect blue sky. You were at peace during those moments. But as we get older, earthly demands start to enter our realm. We want to do well at school, we want to swim well, excel at sports and, of course, please our parents. Gradually, as we forget how to achieve peace, chronic stress enters our body.

SURGEO

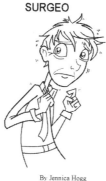

By Jennica Hogg

The Sympathetic Nervous System (Surgeo) is an energy-expanding system. It helps enable the body to deal with stressors, through the flight or fight response. Your heart rate increases, blood pressure goes up, the lungs inflate, the gut is emptied, and blood flow is diverted from the skin to contracted muscles. You are not at peace—you are ready to do battle. If, due to stress, you are in a constant state of readiness, the aging of the body is put into fast forward. And illnesses start to occur.

When the danger trigger or stress passes, the Parasympathetic Nervous System (Peaceo) takes over.

PEACEO

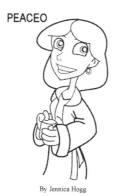

By Jennica Hogg

Its main function is to conserve energy, and promote the quiet and orderly processes of the body. The heart rate decreases, the over-inflated lungs deflate and blood flows back to the gut to allow for absorption of nutrients. Peaceo is associated with peace and tranquility, and hence healing.

It is interesting to note that the Peaceo nerves emerge from the spine bones, only at the neck and tailbone. Growing up, and as adults, we experience the most traumas in our neck and our tailbones. At an early age, minor accidents and poor posture add to the disease of the Parasympathetic Nervous System. In effect, the nerves are "squished", which leads to poor communication in our body computer.

As I worked on my patients, I wanted to find ways to increase the effect of the Peaceo. I knew acupuncture did this to an extent, but I wanted to maximize Peaceo's amazing healing property. My task was to reduce the Surgeo damage and increase the Peaceo healing effect.

1. I learned that it was possible to pull muscle fibers apart which would stop the muscles from wanting to do "Surgeo" (contracted) battle. By placing the muscle fibers in a "C" or "S" shape with the acupuncture needles I was effectively turning off the command for "fight or flight" by making room for the "calcium pump" to work properly. (Muscle contraction is controlled by a calcium pump that must "turn off" in order for muscles to relax. Constant stress prevents this calcium pump from turning off.)[3]

    I found that the muscles quit doing battle and the Parasympathetic Nervous System (Peaceo) took over, allowing the body to experience peace and tranquility. In this restful state, the body's natural de-ager could finally work.

3   D.H. Maclennan, W.J. Rice and N.M. Green (1997) *The mechanism of calcium transport by sacro (endo) plasmic reticulum ca2+ Journal of biological chemistry 272, 28815–28818*

Through this "C-Shape" technique (which you can do on your own), chronic stress can be eliminated in the human body.

2. Another method (which you can also do on your own) is by using your breath. Correct breathing balances the Autonomic Nervous System, and once learned, it is, of course, free! Research for this can be found in the text "Behavioral and Psychological Approaches to Breathing Disorders" edited by Beverly H. Timmons and Ronald Ley.

You will learn how to do these two simple exercises in Chapter Four—"E" is for Exercise.

Chapter Three – F.A.C.E.S.

C is for Costs

In this chapter, I've outlined the average costs of the various anti-aging options available on the market today.

CANADA

EYELID SURGERY $3,000.00–$8,000.00

FACE-LIFT $9,870.00 quoted in British Columbia, Canada (includes GST)

Note: Expenses incurred after March 4, 2010, for purely cosmetic procedures, will not qualify for the medical expense tax credit.

U.S.A.

(Costs appear to be fairly uniform across the U.S.)

EYELID SURGERY $4,000.00–$5,500.00

FACE-LIFT $7,000.00–$9,000.00

U.K.

EYELID SURGERY £2,850.00–£3,600.00 Sterling
    (CDN Dollars equivalent = $5,130.00–$6,480.00)

FACE-LIFT £4,200.00–£5,800.00 Sterling
    (CDN Dollars equivalent = $7,560.00–$10,440.00)

BOTOX AND INJECTABLES (FILLERS)

You must make sure that you are only going to the most highly qualified of practitioners. Botox is stronger than cyanide, so a lot can go wrong. If you are very lucky, you'll get away with $500.00 per visit (more often $700.00 per visit). The recommended treatment cycle is every 3–4 months, but in actual fact, the effects begin to wear off by the end of two.

This, therefore, equates to 6 x $700.00 = $4,200.00 per year.

ACUPUNCTURE ONLY

CANADA

Initial Visit	$65.00–$120.00
Subsequent Visit	$55.00–$120.00

U.S.A.

Initial Visit	$350.00
Subsequent Visit	$225.00
Series of 12	$175.00 per visit

F.A.C.E.S. ACUPUNCTURE
(ACUPUNCTURE, C-SHAPE AND SCRABBLING, AS DEVELOPED BY THE AUTHOR)

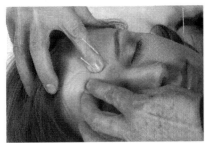

By Kim Elsasser

Initial Visit $350.00
Subsequent Visit $250.00

I am presently taking a limited number of physiotherapists with acupuncture credentials, to teach these techniques. Registered acupuncturists and registered massage therapists will be considered.

Interested candidates, please go to:
www.ConsultEducateTreat.com

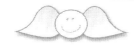

It is highly recommended that individuals aged 30 years or over (depending on the amount of stress, type of diet, etc.) start with a series of 12 sessions of F.A.C.E.S. Acupuncture, with one of the aforementioned qualified practitioners.

You can maintain this by practicing the 5 steps in this book. If you are younger than 30, practicing the 5 steps should be sufficient.

TECHNIQUES LEARNED IN THIS BOOK

SCRABBLING   **FREE**

C-SHAPE   **FREE**

CONNECTIVE TISSUE STRETCH   **FREE**

BREATHING WORK   **FREE**

THE FIVE STEPS   **FREE**

Remember, all five of the F.A.C.E.S. steps improve the health of the face.

Chapter Four – F.A.C.E.S.

E is for Exercises

1. Introduction to *Beauty Without Injections* Facial Exercising
2. Myths
3. What Makes a Wrinkle?
   a. Definition of a Muscle
   b. How a Wrinkle is Made
4. *Beauty Without Injections* Principles for Exercising Facial Muscles
5. INSTRUCTIONS for The Work You Will Do On Your Face:
   a. Scrabbling
   b. C-Shape
      Use both Scrabbling and C-Shape on your:
      i)   Jaw Muscles
      ii) Forehead Muscle
      iii) Cheek Muscles
      iv) Nose Muscles
      v)   Muscles between the Eyebrows
   c. Connective Tissue Stretch
      Use Connective Tissue Stretch:
      i)   Around the Mouth
      ii) At the Temples
      iii) At the Jaw-Line
      iv) At the Corner of the Eyes (Laugh Lines)
6. The Jaw Joints
   Jaw Joint Exercises
7. Posture
   How to Correct Your Posture
8. The Breathe—The Life Force that Controls the Tree of Life
   How to Breathe Properly
9. What If These Steps Seem Too Late?

1. Introduction to *Beauty Without Injections* Facial Exercising
As we all know, exercise is vital to retain the youthful appearance of the body. Education teaches us that the earlier we start—i.e. teens and 20s—and the more we continue, the better we will go through life without weight gain, injuries and diseases. (And of course, we will also have a more youthful, sexy body!) Some have taken this advice; many others have not. The ones who have not, are quite likely suffering by now.

Nothing has changed since the earliest of times:

> *"If we could give every individual the right amount of nourishment and exercise, not too little and not too much, we would have found the safest way to health."* HIPPOCRATES (460–370 B.C.)

Today we are still saying the same thing, but so many are not listening

Who could ask for more than a youthful, sexy body?

Well, actually, the answer to that question is YOU—because by now you should also be thinking about your face! Who could ask for anything more than a youthful, sexy face?

First, let's look at a couple of the myths that are circulating out there regarding the maintenance of the face.

2. Myths
To understand what a myth is, you should know that it is "a widely held, but false belief."

MYTH #1

Muscles get loose and saggy as we age.
Therefore we are bombarded with facial exercises, creams and potions that are actually, in some cases, harmful for the face.
THE TRUTH IS, YOUR FACIAL MUSCLES GET STRINGY *AND TIGHT* (like string with knots in that is pulled almost

to breaking point), CUTTING OFF THE BLOOD AND NERVE FLOW TO YOUR MUSCLES AND SKIN. THIS IS WHAT CAUSES YOUR SKIN TO SAG.

Imagine the effect of 20feet of blood vessels per inch of skin with the flow cut off. To put it another way, look at the flower garden with its beautiful blooms. The hose to water these blooms is 20ft long. If the water is cut off, disaster strikes, because slowly those blooms wither and die.

Think about your poor facial muscles. They are actually working day and night. (THEY MAKE APPROXIMATELY 1,000 REPETITIONS A DAY.) They never get any time off—you grind your teeth at night and produce facial expressions when you dream. THEY DON'T NEED ANY MORE TYPICAL EXERCISE!

MYTH #2

Wrinkles are due to sun damage.

Yes, sun damage *does* kill the top layers of our skin, but this just makes our wrinkles more visible. Wrinkles are actually caused by a totally separate process which I talk about next.

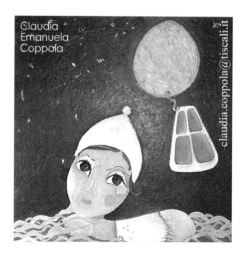

3. What Makes a Wrinkle?

I want to explore how the action of the muscles in the face makes wrinkles.

a. Definition of a Muscle

We have approximately 52 muscles in the face, scalp and above the ears.

To understand more fully, we need to understand what a muscle is.

The word muscle comes from the Latin word *musculus*, meaning LITTLE MOUSE. (I love this term.) A muscle is made of contractile tissue and is derived from the meso dermal layer of embryonic germ cells. Muscles primarily function as a source of power. Smooth muscles are mainly found in our organs, although cardiac muscle—specific to the heart—is striated (grooved). Skeletal muscles (also striated) are a form of fibers that are separated into parallel fibers. These fibers are organized into bands (fibrils) and bundles (fascicles) that contract, to cause the body to move.

Facial muscles can be divided into three types: muscles used for expression, muscles used for chewing, and muscles used for talking.

Look at the difference between your facial muscles and, for example, your shoulder muscles. You will note that your shoulder muscles are able to rest many times during the day when they are not being used. Not so with facial muscles! Facial muscles are a hive of constant activity. They relate to our emotions and are involved in some form of movement day and night. (Take, for instance, the masseter muscle which tenses during the day due to stress and then also during sleep to grind our teeth!) It's no wonder that the face ages faster than the rest of the body.

Also, in relation to the size of the muscles in the body, facial muscles are very small. (Although the exception to this would be some of the muscles found in the hand and foot.)

b. How a Wrinkle is Made

For years we have been told that environmental stress damages our skin. We are told that our skin loses elasticity due to the pollutants in the air, and that damage is done by over-exposure to the sun. That is the smaller truth.

The larger, absolute truth is that wrinkles are formed at right angles to where the muscle fibers run.

OUR FACIAL MUSCLES ARE, IN FACT, THE NUMBER ONE WRINKLE CREATOR:

- Our facial muscles become taut and over-toned as we age because they are in constant movement during the act of chewing, talking, stress, fear and the incessant, ever-changing emotions that show on our face.

- These never-ending contractions eventually cause a substance called "connective tissue" to bind down, PERPENDICULARLY IN THE MUSCLE, which glues the overlying skin to the muscle. It is a revolting concept to comprehend that we actually produce "glue" which eventually forms the "Death-like Mask" of old age!

For example, let's take a look at Orbicularis Oris—the lip muscles:

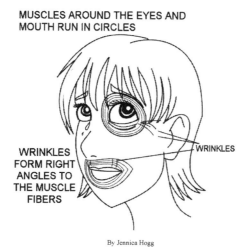

MUSCLES AROUND THE EYES AND
MOUTH RUN IN CIRCLES

WRINKLES
FORM RIGHT
ANGLES TO
THE MUSCLE
FIBERS

WRINKLES

By Jennica Hogg

Smokers form lip lines long before non-smokers, because their lip muscles are worked to exhaustion.

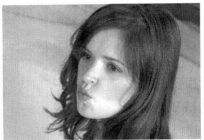

By Kim Elsasser

So, to reverse the aging process, we need to release our facial muscles, and the connective tissue that is gluing our muscles to our face, forming wrinkles.

Facial muscles never rest

They say we have approximately 60,000 thoughts a day running through our mind, and probably these same thoughts will repeat the next day. People often feel that to have a constant stream of chatter in the brain is normal. (It's called the monkey brain.) But if each one of these thoughts produces an emotion, then each thought will produce some facial movement.

Therefore, if you can engage in some form of meditation— say, yoga—you will stop the traffic-flow through your mind, which will in turn decrease the emotion-related activity of your facial muscles so they can finally rest.

Perhaps you have followed Eckhart Tolle's "A New Earth" on the Oprah Winfrey Show, where he talks about staying in the present moment by focusing on the breath. This also quietens the mind, which in turn has a softening (de-aging) effect on the face.

And this is also where facial acupuncture comes into play. Facial acupuncture causes the facial muscles to relax by inserting a thin needle into the muscle knot (trigger point) to relax the point of increased hyper-irritability. Relaxation can be further enhanced by placing the facial muscle into a C-Shape—which you can do on your own, as I'll discuss later.

4. *Beauty Without Injections* Principles for Exercising Facial Muscles

1. Wrinkles are formed at right angles to how the muscle fibers run.

2. The muscles of the face have become over-toned. This is contrary to the popular belief that aging in the face and sagging skin is due to *loss* of tone.

   To understand this, look at the calves of a long-distance runner—they are fibrous and taut. They are over-toned.

   In the face, you want to restore your muscles to a relaxed full-ness and length, and fill out your skin with softened, plump, well-fleshed muscles.

   Think of these taut facial muscles as short ropes with a knot in the middle. You would know that, by pulling on either end, it will make the rope longer—but the knot is still there. The following exercises will show you how to undo this knot so that you can control the normal length and softness of your muscles.

3. If you do the classic facial exercises, these will make wrinkles worse.

   For example, pucker the mouth. This will make lip lines worse. (This is why smokers always have pronounced lip lines.)

4. As the face does its thousands of repetitive little movements every day, and we start to age, the connective tissue sur-rounding every muscle fiber begins to act like glue and helps in forming lines. As you examine your face, you will find not only lines, but also areas where the skin does not move freely anymore. (For example, the skin on the forehead.)

5. INSTRUCTIONS for The Work You Will Do On Your Face:

a. Scrabbling (Definition—means to run quickly across. For example, "The crabs scrabbled across the rocks.")

This exercise will help prevent the binding-down of connective tissue on your wrinkles. This binding-down blocks the free flow of toxins in the lymphatic system of your face. These toxins should flow from the mid-line of your face, out to your ear, and be disposed of in the jugular vein.

<u>To Perform Scrabbling</u>:
Gently pick up the skin between the thumb and second and third fingers, and roll toward the ear. In some areas there will be resistance; do not force, just gently roll. This will get better with time.

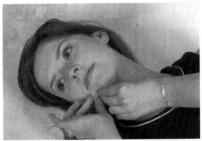

By Kim Elsasser

(I have also found that doing this from the jaw bone up, is very beneficial.)

b. C-Shape

This exercise is applied to the face in order to relax the over-toned facial muscles. When the muscles are too tight in the face, they block the blood and nerve flow, as well as the flow of lymph mentioned in "Scrabbling" above.

To Perform the C-Shape Exercise:

Place one or two fingers (whichever is more comfortable) from one hand, directly above one or two fingers from your other hand, and sink them toward the skull until you feel resistance below. Push one hand one way, and the other in the opposite direction. YOU HAVE CREATED A "C-SHAPE." If done correctly, you should feel a sharp sensation. This is the movement of the connective tissue releasing the tight, taut band of muscle.

The calcium pump in your muscles is now free, allowing your muscles to relax. With the relaxation of the over-toned muscles, blood flows freely, to and from the face, and nerve transmission goes unimpeded.

This exercise evolved in the late 1920s, when a physiotherapist in Germany called Elizabeth Dicke was suffering a fatal circulatory condition and had been put into a back room of the hospital to die. She started to perform "soft tissue" massage on herself, and noticed a sharp sensation followed by a feeling of warmth. She completely recovered, and ten years of research later, she set up a teaching protocol for physiotherapy students in Germany.

In the 1980s, a British physiotherapist, Jacqueline Flexney-Briscoe, studied in Germany and brought it back to Britain. At the same time, a physiotherapist called John Barnes was teaching Myofascial Release in the United States, which was also based on this connective tissue release.

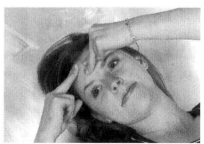

By Kim Elsasser

Perform Scrabbling and C-Shape Exercises on the Following Facial Muscles:

i) Jaw Muscles

Do dark circles and bags under your eyes bother you? Dr. Travell states that this might be due to the muscles around the jaw joint (temporalis, masseter, pterygoid) becoming tight bands.[4]

These bands cut off the blood flow from under the eye and above the ear by blocking the vein which drains the area under the eye, and hence causing dark circles and bags. Using the Scrabbling and C-Shape exercises will release this tension in the jaw.

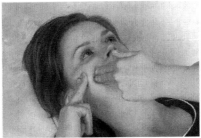

By Kim Elsasser

This group of muscles runs from the outer corner of the jaw, up to the cheek bone at the outer corner of the eye. Wrinkles produced are the jowl lines.

ii) Forehead Muscle

This muscle (frontalis) starts above the eyebrows and extends about an inch into the scalp. The muscle fibers run vertically and therefore the wrinkles are horizontal across the forehead. This muscle is the one that's most frequently Botoxed.

---

4 *Pg. 227, 228 Myofascial Pain and Dysfunction, Janet G. Travell, M.D.; David G. Simons, M.D.*

iii) Cheek Muscles

These muscles run from the outer corner of the mouth and up to the cheek bone at the outer corner of the eye. Wrinkles produced are the grooves that run from the nose to the corners of the mouth (naso labia line).

iv) Nose Muscles

There are several muscles that run from the lip, up to the nose or the eye muscle. These produce the lines around the nose when you contract your nose in disgust.

v) Muscles between the Eyebrows

These tiny muscles (gabellar) produce the frown lines between the eyebrows. They can start contracting at a very early age.

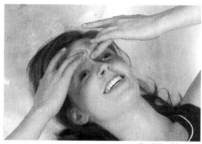

By Kim Elsasser

c. Connective Tissue Stretch

This exercise is applied to the following areas of the face to gently release the binding-down around the facial lines:

i) Around the Mouth

Place a finger in each corner of your mouth.
Gently stretch outwards until you feel resistance.
Hold for 1½ to 3 minutes.
You might feel a burn in certain areas around your mouth—

this is where connective tissue is gluing down to form wrinkles.

Wait for the release of the connective tissue (glue), which will feel like the whoosh of going down a slide.

This prevents the vertical lip lines.

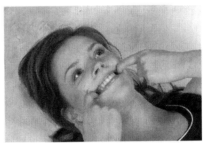

By Kim Elsasser

ii) At the Temples

Place three fingers at the end of an eyebrow.

Sink them gently until you meet with resistance.

Gently push the resistance up.

Hold for 1½ to 3 minutes.

You will feel a gentle release.

This helps prevent laugh lines but also helps to lift the eyebrows.

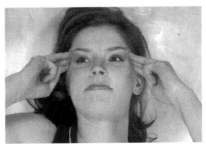

By Kim Elsasser

iii) At the Jaw-Line

Place your fingers on your jaw-line, just under your mouth, and push toward your ear.
Wait for the resistance.
Hold for the 1½ to 3 minutes.
Wait for a release.

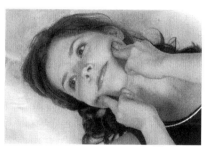

By Kim Elsasser

iv) At the Corner of the Eyes (Laugh Lines)

Place one finger of one hand slightly above the outer corner of your eye.
Place another finger from the other hand slightly below the outer corner of the same eye.
Gently stretch; you will feel the characteristic burn. Wait for the gentle release.

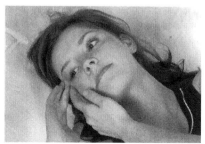

By Kim Elsasser

6. The Jaw Joints

Experts agree that the jaw joints are the most complex and mysterious joints in the body. They are located on either side of the head, just in front of the ears.

The structures that make it possible to open and close the mouth are very specialized; they work together when you chew, speak, express emotions and swallow. These structures include 5 pairs of muscles, ligament, bone and joints.

The jaw joints have two functions:

1. The hinge movement.
2. The side-to-side movement.

It is common knowledge that we must keep up the movement of the joints of the body in general as we age or we lose the ability to move.

MOBILITY is equated with YOUTHFULNESS

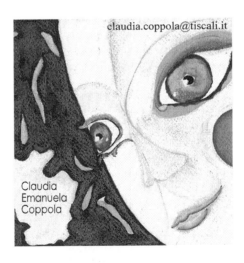

The jaw joints also stiffen as we age, giving the appearance of narrowing, or aging, of the jaw. (In plastic surgery, this is one area they can't correct. A face-lift will just pull loose skin up over a narrowed jaw.)

This stiffening of the jaw joints is further compounded by tightening of the jaw *muscles*—temporalis, masseter and the pterygoids—which happens, as we've discussed, through constant activity or stress. (Remember how, in Chapter Two, stress sets off "SURGEO" which causes the muscles to contract.)

Angel Wing Test

To see if your jaw muscles have tightened, place your hands on your cheek bones in front of your ears. Slide them above and below the cheek bones. If you find dents, your "angel wings have stopped flying" (the jaw muscles have shortened and tightened—you are getting older). Techniques to release these jaw muscles are discussed under the Scrabbling and C-Shape exercise section, point i).

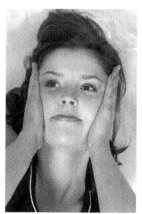

By Kim Elsasser

It is interesting to note that the jaw joints (temporomandibular joints) are the location of an intersection in acupuncture of three major energy meridians—the stomach, the small intestine and the san jaou meridians. Relief of jaw joint dysfunction can spark a tremendous healing process in the body.

It is estimated that up to 25% of the population suffers

from a jaw disorder—with a large percentage affected being younger people.[5] This is a much larger percentage than for other joint disorders. I believe this is related to stress (affecting the jaw *muscles*), and also the lack of regular exercise given to the actual *joints*. Everyone is off to yoga, soccer and pole-walking to exercise the joints in their body, but they forget about the joints in their face. The following simple jaw joint exercises can be done anywhere:

a. **Jaw Joint Exercises**
(I'm not in favor of doing activities such as chewing because we have to do a lot of that every day. I prefer a full range of motion, but by this I mean only moving the joint as far as you can in *one direction at a time*, without putting undue stress on it.)

Exercise 1
Open your jaw joint (mouth) as far as you can without causing yourself pain or stress. (A general rule of thumb for a healthy opening is: Can you place three fingers vertically in your mouth?)

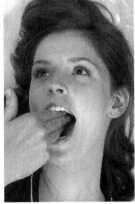

By Kim Elsasser

5   *Hedge V. A review of the disorders of the temporomandibular joint, J Indian Prosthodont Soc (serial online) 2005 (cited 2008, Jun 14); 5:56–61*

You can use a finger from either hand to gently assist with the opening. Hold for 1½ to 3 minutes.

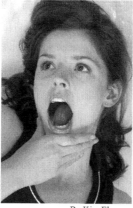

By Kim Elsasser

Again, wait for that gentle release which is the connective tissue (glue) releasing. Make sure that you are maintaining the correct posture while performing this exercise. Relax, breathe into the abdomen. Note the relaxation as you breathe out.

Exercise 2

Gently open your mouth. Glide your jaw, first to one side. Apply gentle, sustained pressure for 1½ to 3 minutes. Repeat on the other side.

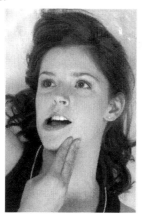

By Kim Elsasser

Exercise 3

Gently open your mouth. Now move your lower teeth (jaw) forward until they are in front of your upper teeth (protraction). There is a tendency for our lower jaw to move backwards as time goes by, as well as for the jaw joints to stiffen generally.

Performing these three simple exercises may prevent painful temporomandibular joint (T.M.J.) disorders, as well as slow down the aging and narrowing of the jaw-line which produces the long and horsy look.

7. Posture

LEAD WITH THE HEART AND NOT THE HEAD

Meet Mr. L.W. THANTH.

(**L**—Lead, **W**—With,
T—The, **H**—Heart, **A**—And, **N**—Not, **T**—The, **H**—Head)

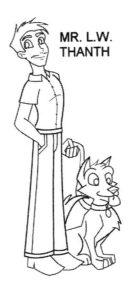

MR. L.W. THANTH

By Jennica Hogg

Not only is "Mr. L.W. THANTH" good for spiritual balancing, this amazing man also helps balance the physical body. For posture correction, all you need to think about is "Mr. L.W. THANTH," add a lift toward the sky, and your body will fall into alignment.

Over the years as a physiotherapist, I have observed that people who do not have proper alignment appear as beaten dogs, with their tails curled between their legs. I call it the POSTURE OF SUBMISSION.

They achieve this by:

1. Curving their lower tailbone under.

2. This rounds their upper and lower back.

3. Their chest collapses inward.

4. Their shoulders round forward and go up under their ears.

5. Their head juts forward and their chin falls down.

**BAD POSTURE
OF SUBMISSION**

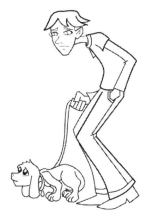

By Jennica Hogg

This makes three things clear:

i. The emotional connection to posture is blatant.

ii. If the chest gets compressed, then the person can't breathe and is basically suffocating.

iii. With poor posture, the chin compacts downward towards the chest, producing folds under the chin—or the "double chin."

In summary, improper posture takes its toll on the body and face.

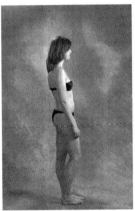

By Kim Elsasser

As mentioned in Chapter Two, the calming "PEACEO" nerves for the Tree of Life come from the neck spine bones and the tailbone. With poor posture, added pressure is put on the nerves as they emerge from the spine bones, making it more difficult for "PEACEO" to attain balance.

As soon as you sit, practice doing the "Mr. L.W. THANTH" with a lift. Also do the same when standing.

How to Correct Your Posture:

1. Relax the shoulders, bringing them down and away from the ears. Pull your blades down the back of your chest wall.

2. Bring your chest out.

3. Your ears should be in alignment with your shoulders and hips.

4. Pull your abs toward your spinal column.

5. Pull your pelvic floor up.

6. MOST IMPORTANTLY, lift your whole body up. Take off and soar, as you were meant to do in this life!

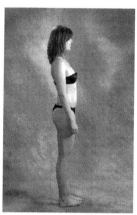

By Kim Elsasser

8. The Breathe—The Life Force that Controls the Tree of Life
JUST AS THERE IS A RIGHT AND A WRONG WAY TO EAT, SO THERE IS A RIGHT AND A WRONG WAY TO BREATHE.

Most North Americans, due to their high levels of stress, either breathe too quickly and too shallowly, or hold their breath. When you see someone yawning excessively, or sighing, it indicates that they are not getting enough oxygen. They are breathing with the muscles around their necks and shoulders in a pattern called hyperventilation.[6]

6 *Emedicine Hyperventilation Syndrome: Article by Edward J. Newton, M.D., FACEP, FRCPC*

Healthy Breathing
I am only concerned about getting the air down to where it belongs. You will find many different explanations of how to do this, but I will explain the simplest method.

I want you to visualize a puppy that is sleeping. Look at its little belly, rising and falling. It looks so relaxed. This is called "diaphragmatic breathing."

When you breathe this way, you use the large parachute-shaped muscle (the diaphragm) that attaches to your lower ribs. It bellows up and down when you are breathing into your belly.

Most people will go a lifetime never connecting with this muscle, which is tragic because, not only are they depleting their bodies of the proper oxygen mixture (see Article cited in footnote on previous page), but in eastern medicine, one of the major energy centers is located just below the belly button. Also, just as with other muscles in the body, if not used it will shrivel away.

How to Breathe Properly:

1. Sitting or lying comfortably, bring that incredible, life-giving substance in through your nose.

2. At the same time, make sure that your neck and shoulders are not rising and that they are completely relaxed. (Raising your neck and shoulders indicates that you are using your accessory muscles to breathe—hyperventilation.)

3. Notice the air as it passes down through your throat.

4. Next, feel the air in your chest.

5. You will feel your ribs expand.

6. Now, like the puppy, you will feel your belly expand. This is the action of the diaphragm muscle expanding down to bring the air in—just like the sail of a boat.

7. Hold that expansion—it should feel so good.

8. Finally, just relax, and on its own, the air will flow out like the wind.

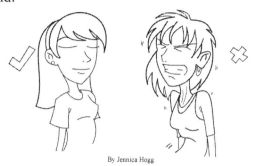

By Jennica Hogg

It is common knowledge that by following this "PUPPY" breathing, not only will your muscles relax, but there will be a whole relaxation of the body.

9. What If These Steps Seem Too Late?

It is never, ever too late to turn around the health of your body and face. Remember how, in my youth, I struggled with my health and weight? It took several decades before I was able to adopt a truly healthy lifestyle, but I have benefited tremendously since then.

There might be instances when healthy living simply isn't enough—for example, say, a man who has stayed in shape all his life, but who has a worn-out, painful right knee. The wise thing in this case would be to accept medical help. We live in amazing times, and a life-enhancing knee replacement would take the pain away.

But in general terms, healthy living, exercise and a regard for our natural bodies, are all that's needed to improve fitness one-hundred-fold, and regain our youthful looks.

I have kept for many years, the study published by Anthony A. Vandervoort, P.T., University of Western Ontario, where he demonstrates that the muscle system is reversible even in the very frail and elderly.

Chapter Five – F.A.C.E.S.

S is for Skin

The skin is the largest organ in our bodies. This always catches people by surprise—generally we know that our kidneys and lungs are organs, but not our skin. Is it because we can see skin with the naked eye and all our other organs are hidden UNDER the skin?

Stand in front of your refrigerator. For most people, their skin and body will take up about 1/8 to 1/4 of the cubic size of their refrigerator. Instead of holding and protecting food, your skin covers and protects everything inside your body, acting like a shield of armor to keep out diseases and water, and controlling your body temperature.

Your skin also stops your other organs, muscles and bones from hanging out all over the place!

Skin has nerve endings which provide information, control evaporation, and play a part in synthesis, etc.

Layers

The skin is made up of three layers:

1. Epidermis Layer

For those of us who are concerned about healthy skin, this is where all the action takes place.

When we look at skin, we see the top of the epidermis. However, what we are actually looking at is dead skin. (We carry around 25 to 30 layers of dead skin.)

Considered in this light, the skin can suddenly seem quite repulsive, especially as it looks fine to the naked eye!

When we are young and healthy, we slough off our dead skin

and replace it with new skin naturally. The epidermis acts like a factory. New skin cells form at the bottom of the epidermis layer, and when they are ready, they start heading for the skin's surface to take the place of the dying or dead cells near the top. This trip, in a healthy person, takes from 2 weeks to a month.

As we reach our 30s, or lose optimum health, this natural sloughing process slows—and this is how skin cancers begin.

2. Dermis Layer
Lying beneath the epidermis, the dermis layer of the skin consists of connective tissue.

This connective tissue is the material that "lays down and binds" in the wrinkle formation—at 90 degrees to the muscle fiber.

3. Hypodermis Layer
This layer lies below the dermis—attaching the skin to underlying bone and muscle, and supplying it with blood vessels and nerves.

Again, the connective tissue in this layer, binds and glues down perpendicularly to the direction of the muscle fibers, basically forming scar tissue.

Returning to the epidermis... Remember when you are eying up the outside of your refrigerator, trying to picture the size of your skin, it is actually dead skin you are looking at.

Years ago, did you ever go to the Midway or the fair? There was an exhibit called the "Freak Show," where individuals with an unusual disability would be put on display so that everyone could be "repulsed." (This title shows how far people with disabilities have come in regaining their dignity.) You'd see the four-hundred-pound lady; the lady covered with all kinds of facial hair so that she looked like a man; and the "alligator" lady—an unfortunate individual with an exaggeration of the normal 25–30 layers of dead skin.

Hopefully this will encourage you to look into the more advanced methods of exfoliation for your own skin!

Getting Rid Of Dead Skin

Everyone takes for granted that teeth should be cleaned 2 to 3 times a day, and that a dental hygienist should be seen, say 2 or 3 times a year. (This went up a notch when teeth cleaning kits came out.) And of course, everyone regularly visits their dentist to make sure that their teeth are healthy.

Is it not sensible, therefore, to suggest that cleansing of the skin should go way beyond simple soap and water?

Between the ages of 20 and 30, people should start thinking in terms of accelerating their slowing skin cell turnover. A TRIP TO THEIR DERMATOLOGIST (A DOCTOR WHO SPECIALIZES IN THE STUDY OF THE SKIN) WILL PUT THEM ON THE BEST PROGRAM TO EXFOLIATE THOSE 25–30 LAYERS OF DEAD SKIN AT A NORMAL RATE. THIS, COMBINED WITH THE FIVE-STEP "BEAUTY WITHOUT INJECTIONS" PROGRAM, WILL PRODUCE AMAZING SKIN. (IN PLASTIC SURGEON'S OFFICES THEY ALSO HAVE EXCELLENT NURSES WHO HAVE SPECIALIZED IN THE CARE OF THE SKIN.)

Practicing the five-step program and visiting a dermatologist will be up there alongside mammograms and pap smear tests because you are now definitely preventing skin cancer. (An unwanted side effect to the build-up of dead cells is skin cancer, which is now on the increase.)

My Routine

As pointed out earlier, I started Retin-A in my thirties, when it first became available. It was to be touted as the most beneficial product for the skin that had come out in decades—and it certainly accelerates skin cell turnover. But it is not for everyone, and dermatologists soon found themselves inundated with patients who were suffering from red and irritated skin after using it. I was fortunate—I have always been able to tolerate Retin-A—although I only use it in the winter, as it makes skin more sensitive to the sun. Over the last 20 years I have alternated Retin-A with 10% glycolic acid on my face and body, which has worked very well for me. (Again though, 10% glycolic acid is not for everyone, and will be way too harsh for more sensitive skins. Only your specialist can advise you.)

The Emotions And The Skin
For centuries, people have linked emotions to skin—intuitively knowing, before there was medical evidence, that our emotional wellbeing affects the quality of our skin.

Look at the sayings that go back generations:

• It's only skin deep;
• You need to toughen up that skin of yours.

From Chapter Two we now know that there is a computer in our body (*the Autonomic Nervous System (A.N.S.)* or *Tree of Life*), that works day and night, without our conscious control, trying to keep vital functions in balance. We also know that a very poor job is being made of it, leading to illnesses and, of course, aging.

If we think about the skin specifically, there is far too much stress, fear and negative "monkey brain" going on in our lives. Which means there is too much "SURGEO" (the Sympathetic Nervous System which kicks into fight or flight mode in response to stress), which in turn means blood is being diverted away from the skin and internal organs, and is being sent to the muscles, brain and heart TO DO BATTLE. Not good news for our skin!

The vast majority of researchers still feel that the Autonomic Nervous System (A.N.S.) is an involuntary process, and therefore out of our control.

But this is not true.

Refer back to Chapter Two. A certain amount of conscious control can be exerted over the Autonomic Nervous System, demonstrated by yoga and zen buddhism, for example. The most obvious drawback to these two practices is that they require great discipline. Alternatives are acupuncture, the C-Shape and Breathing exercises outlined in Chapter Four, laughter, eating healthy foods…in fact, anything that brings peace to your soul.

Restoring peace and balance to your system will shunt blood-flow back to your skin. THE BATTLE WILL BE OVER. Plump skin versus shriveled skin IS controllable!

The choice is yours. Do you want…

PLUMP
LUMINOUS
GLOWING
SMOOTH SKIN

or

SHRIVELED
DRY
HANGING
CELLULITE?

To Recap:

In today's society, the Autonomic Nervous System is sick. In order to get your healthy computer back and regenerate your skin, you need to increase the "PEACEO" healing effect. Think of Peaceo (the peaceful Parasympathetic Nervous System) as the mouse on your computer system at home. You carefully navigate with your mouse, deleting possible viruses in e-mails, calmly downloading specific tools to increase protection, backing up the computer, etc. The mouse is at the head of the quiet and orderly processes of your computer, just as Peaceo controls the quiet and orderly processes of your body's computer to trigger your healing and protection.

Remember, your skin is your body's largest organ and it needs looking after.

Think of your skin as your finest dress or suit—the one article of clothing that, when you put it on, makes you feel you are the sexiest, hottest, most attractive person in the whole world.

The clothing will only fit well and look its best if the body is healthy.

To have healthy skin, you need to nourish it from both the outside and the inside.

"BEAUTY WITHOUT INJECTIONS" is the first book to demonstrate this, helping you find health, happiness, and the face and body you had 10–20 years ago. Five steps that require no expensive lotions or procedures and that give the empowerment to you, my dear reader.

With this supreme health we can go out and help the less fortunate.

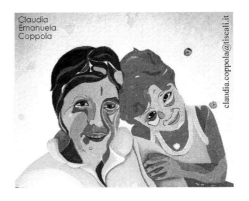

Every morning when I wake up, I repeat the following mantra which resonates very deeply with me:

> *As long as space endures and sentient beings remain, may I too remain to ease the sufferings of this world.*

Mahatma Gandhi said: "True world healing will only happen when each individual goes within and heals themselves."

All my love to you.

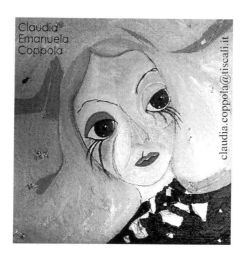

About the Author

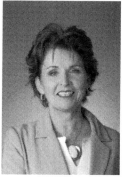

By Eric's Photography

HELEN ELIZABETH DAY P.T. (Physiotherapy)
C.A.F.C.I. (Acupuncture)

Helen E. Day was born in Edmonton, Alberta, Canada into a professional family with an orthopedic surgeon father and a dietician mother.

She graduated from the University of Alberta, School of Physiotherapy in 1969. In 1981 she returned to University to increase her knowledge and skills.

In 1992, she graduated from North America's first University level School of Acupuncture. She moved, with her daughter, in 1993 to Kelowna, B.C., and opened her own private practice.

In the past decade she has educated herself on the works of Dr. Janet Travell, President Kennedy's personal physician.

Her research into using acupuncture on trigger points led to the discovery that, not only was the patient's pain relieved in the affected area, but it also looked younger.

She taught at Okanagan University College (now known as Okanagan College) in 2000 and 2001.

In May of 2002, during simple bladder surgery, she went into pre-cardiac arrest. The alert nurses gave her an injection that saved her life, but unfortunately left her with five years of constant pain, due to spinal cord injury to the inside of the spinal column, affecting sensory nerves and leading to constant neuropathic (nerve) pain known as arachnoiditis. Dr. J. Antonio Aldrete, M.D., M.S., wrote the book "Arachnoiditis: The Silent Epidemic."

During her recovery, she began to treat herself three to four times a week using the steps outlined in this book. The results were amazing, and by 2007, she was able to resume her work on a limited basis.

She is presently working on her new non-fiction book on chronic, persistent pain, called "When Good People Have To Lie." Also the fiction fantasy, "Tringaling and The Land Of The Wakens"—a tale with an incredible lesson to teach, about a turtle, seal, and blue and gold macaw, who are all stranded on a small rock in the ocean. The aged seal has the ancient knowledge to access the Waken kingdom, under the waves, where only peace reigns...

Index

99

Also by Helen E. Day:

"CREAM"—AN ANTI-AGING MIRACLE

I made this cream when I was injured, using it daily for many years over my injured lumbar spinal bones and on the muscles on either side. All-natural, its many success stories (apart from my own) include:

"For many years I had a persistent fungus infection under my toenails, especially on my left foot. Over time, the nails became distorted, thickened and discolored. Nothing that I tried helped. Helen suggested that I try nightly applications of her anti-aging skin cream "CREAM" while wearing a thin cotton sock to protect the bedding. THERE WAS AN IMMEDIATE IMPROVEMENT in the appearance and color of my toes. Gradually the misshapen and discolored nails grew out and the new ones are healthy and strong." Robby D., 89, Summerland, B.C., Canada
NOTE: For very resistant toe nail fungus, try acupuncture to the corner of the toe nail beds (Jing well points), in addition to "CREAM" applied nightly.

"I would like to tell you about the extraordinary results I had using Helen Day's anti-aging cream. For two years I had a growth on my right inner thigh. My doctor removed it 3 times but it always grew back again. It was very uncomfortable because it would catch on my clothing and open and bleed. Helen suggested that I try this skin cream she had developed. I put it on daily and within a month the growth was gone. I can't recommend "CREAM" too highly." Winnie L., 91, Kelowna, B.C., Canada

"I use the facial formulation of "CREAM". It is out of this world for results. I combine it with C-Shape and Scrabbling, and for the first time in years I could see the blood flow in my skin. My skin absolutely glows." C.H., Vancouver, B.C., Canada

Sold in 50ml bottles
1 bottle: $60.00 Canadian Dollars
2–4 bottles: $50.00 Canadian Dollars each
5 bottles or more: $45.00 Canadian Dollars each
To Order, Phone: 1-250-448-0438
Or Write To: 773-2 Stockwell Avenue, Kelowna
British Columbia, Canada V1Y 6W1

Notes

Notes

Notes

Notes

The Paintings of Claudia Emanuela Coppola

CLAUDIA EMANUELA COPPOLA, born in Milano, Italy in 1966, is uniquely positioned as an artist, moving effortlessly across disciplines as a writer, painter, theatre director and illustrator. Sinuous lines, vivid colors and sensational tones are characteristic of the faces she paints. Trapped in their dreamy world, Coppola's figures have the power to open us to the soul with their glance. Coppola has been widely recognized with publications, awards and exhibitions in New York, Miami, Budapest, Paris, London, Milano, Roma, Genova, Chianciano, Madrid, Taormina, Treviso and Venezia.

Contact:

claudia.coppola@tiscali.it
www.claudiaemanuelacoppola.ning.com

To Look At The Painting Works:

http://www.youtube.com/watch?v=Dq7G396522E

Made in the USA
Charleston, SC
15 November 2013